Practice Management Compendium

T0233679

Part 3: Finance and Reports

Practice Management Compendium

Part 1: Understanding the Contract
Part 2: Organising the Practice
Part 3: Finance and Reports
Part 4: Clinical Practices

Practice Management Compendium

Part 3: Finance and Reports

by

John Fry

and

Kenneth Scott
General Practitioners

and

Pauline Jeffree
Practice Nurse,
Beckenham, Kent

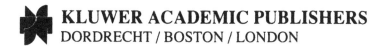
KLUWER ACADEMIC PUBLISHERS
DORDRECHT / BOSTON / LONDON

Distributors

for the United States and Canada : Kluwer Academic Publishers, P.O. Box 358, Accord Station, Hingham, MA 02018-0358, U.S.A.
for all other countries : Kluwer Academic Publishers Group, Distribution Center, P.O. Box 322, 3300 AH Dordrecht, The Netherlands.

ISBN 0-7923-8943-3

Published in the United Kingdom by Kluwer Academic Publishers, P.O. Box 55, Lancaster, U.K.

Kluwer Academic Publishers BV incorporates the publishing programmes of D. Reidel, Martinus Nijhoff, Dr W. Junk and MTP Press.

Origination by Roby Education Ltd, Liverpool.

Printed in Gt. Britain by Butler and Tanner Ltd., Frome and London.

Contents

Foreword

General Practice is undergoing the most major series of changes since the introduction of the National Health Service in 1948. They concern both concepts of care and practical details of the way care is delivered. In spite of the hostility generated by the changes most of the broad general concepts have been accepted. The principle of patients having more choice is widely supported, the inclusion of preventive medicine and anticipatory care in the responsibilities of practice has few opponents, the introduction of audit as a way of improving performance has been generally welcomed. Even the idea of putting GPs in better financial management of patients and drug budgets has had supporters in principle. The antipathy has generally related to the method of introduction of these changes. One important concern has been the time requirements of the New Contract and the feeling that these will erode the real nature of our work: the close personal relationship with patients.

If we improve the quality of our management this is less likely to happen. We shall be able to work within the New Contract and retain the quality of service we provide. If we improve the understanding of our staff of what we are trying to achieve we are more likely to reach the targets that we set whilst keeping people happy.

This book sets out to explain the New Contract. An understanding of this will be essential to those of us who have to work the system, and if we are better informed it will give us more chance of making the sensible amendments that will certainly be needed. I believe it will be a highly valuable source of information for Principals, Trainees and staff in practice and very strongly commend it.

Professor Sir Michael Drury
Head, Department of General Practice
University of Birmingham Medical School

Chapter 1

Clinical Goals and Challenges

HEALTH CARE - TODAY AND TOMORROW

There is no perfect health care system anywhere in the world. All countries face similar problems, dilemmas and frustrations.

There is everywhere an insoluble equation of being unable to match "wants" and "needs" with "available resources". It is very evident that there are finite limits as to how much can be spent by providers, be they governments, insurance bodies or private individuals. Inevitably this must lead to rationing and, in turn, this creates problems of controls and directives and various ways of trying to obtain "value for money".

Another current debate concerns ways of improving quality of life through more quantity of medical care, and this in turn has to be related to the stark limitations of even the most advanced medical technologies. It is clear that a major factor in achieving and maintaining health of the people lies in the standards of social amenities such as good housing, safe environment, employment, adequate income to pay for luxuries, as well as life's essentials.

...there are finite limits as to how much can be spent by providers...

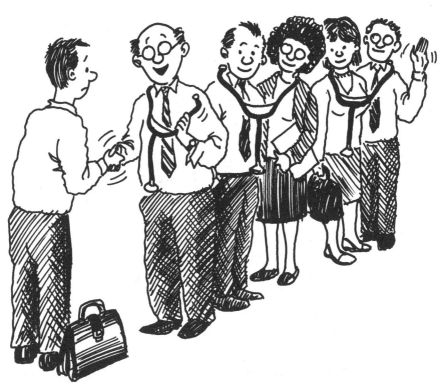

"Welcome to the team. Oh, and by the way, as we have only one stethoscope between us you'll be on a party line."

It has to be realistically accepted that there are, and always will be, major social and health inequalities. We are not born equal, nor do we die equal. However, any good health care system must endeavour to provide equal opportunities for receiving appropriate care.

Today in the United Kingdom we are reasonably healthy, as assessed by the traditional health indices of infant and maternal mortalities, and life expectancies. Yet there are many who die long before they should from preventable diseases and situations. In theory all accidents are preventable and so are some of the early deaths in the 40s, 50s and 60s from heart diseases, strokes and cancers.

...we are not born equal...

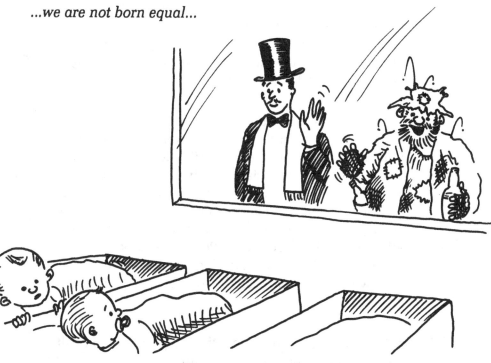

"I hope my dad's the one on the left!"

When it comes to social amenities and social pathologies, we do less well in world comparisons, with one-third of adults still smoking; diets that are unbalanced in food and in excess of alcohol; environmental pollution that can lead to a spectrum of possible life threatening conditions; lack of regular exercise; and poor conditions at work and at home.

Tomorrow has to be concerned as much, if not more, with "prevention" as with "cure" of disease.

However, there are two provisos that have to be realistically appreciated before we lose our sense of balance and common-sense:

- How much is preventable and what measures are effective and beneficial? It is worse than useless to direct all GPs to undertake screening unless there is evidence that it will lead to better health and longer life . It may be that some preventive procedures are better than others, but this has to be researched and implemented.

- What should be the responsibilities of the various participants in the business of health care? The people (public and patients) have responsibilities as well as health professionals and politicians. Individuals must accept responsibilities for health attainment and maintenance and disease prevention. Professionals such as doctors, nurses and others must use available resources efficiently, effectively and economically. Politicians, or other providers of health resources, must be prepared to meet costs whenever possible and avoid unnecessary directives and controls.

Ultimately, there has to be a realistic mirage of a good health care system which, although never quite attainable, should be strived for.

It is worth reminding ourselves that good care by good doctors must be personal care on a one-to-one relationship, even in a team, and endeavour to - "cure sometimes, relieve often, comfort always, prevent hopefully".

PLACE OF GENERAL PRACTICE (primary health care)

In all health systems, whatever their form, there are 4 inevitable levels of care relating to similar population bases and administrative organisation, in countries of like development. Here it has to be noted that the form and structure of a national health system evolve through historical, social and economic factors. Thus, the British National Health Service was not new and revolutionary when it began in 5 July 1948. It had evolved through almost a century of sick funds, friendly societies and other pre-paid voluntary insurance schemes and National Health Insurance for lower paid workers.

The 4 levels of care (Figure 1.1) are -

- Self care by individuals and families
- Primary professional care, including general practice with direct access to patients.
- Secondary general specialist care by generalist surgeons, physicians, OBG, paediatricians, orthopaedists, psychiatrists and others working from a district general hospital, to whom patients are referred by general practitioners.
- Tertiary super-specialist care by regional units such as cardiac surgery, neurology, transplantation work and others.

General practice in UK traditionally has been the major source of primary professional care and this was incorporated into the structure of the NHS in 1948, and maintained

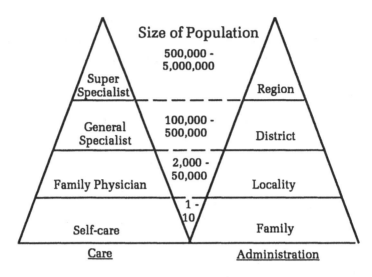

Fig. 1.1 Levels of care

since. Now there are other sources of primary professional care by paramedical workers, but GPs are the only ones who can refer patients to specialists and hospitals.

FEATURES OF GENERAL PRACTICE

General practice in NHS has the following features -

- Direct access to GP (or deputy) by NHS registered patients on a 24 hour basis requiring effective and efficient organisation.
- First contact care, meaning that the GP is brought packages of undefined problems and symptoms by patients which he/she has to untie, unravel, diagnose and manage, as well as sort out. Quite different from the pre-packaged sectorised and categorised groups seen at

specialist clinics. The GP has to be a good diagnostician, therapist and manager.

- Long term and continuing care: most patients remain under the care of their GP for many years and in our relatively stable society GPs are privileged to care for patients over 20, 30 or 40 years. It is not unusual to look after 4 generations of a family at any time - great-granny, granny, mother and infant. Such long term associations offer particular opportunities to develop good, continuing doctor-patient and personal and family relationships.

- Small and static population base: at present, on average, a GP has around 2,000 NHS patients and a group practice of 5 GPs will have 10,000 patients.

- The disease spectrum in general practice is very different from that of hospital practice. Inevitably, because the GP is the doctor-of-first-contact caring for a population of 2000, the clinical spectrum will be that expected in a population of this size with a preponderance of common minor and chronic disorders, rather than the selected cases seen in hospitals. The GP has to become expert in understanding the nature, outcome and significance of these conditions and organise appropriate management. This is difficult because of lack of reliable research data on natural history and clinical trials.

The clinical content of general practice (Tables 1.1 - 1.4) shows the expected annual numbers of cases of various conditions that can be expected in an average size practice.

Table 1.1 Chronic disesse

	Annual persons consulting	
	per 2,500	per 10,000
High blood pressure	100	400
Chronic rheumatism (arthritis)	100	400
Chronic psychiatric problems	75	300
Ischaemic heart disease	50	200
Obesity	50	200
Cardiac failure	20	80
Anaemia	30	120
Cancers (under care)	30	120
Asthma	40	160
Diabetes	20	80
Varicose veins	30	120
Peptic ulcers	25	100
Strokes	20	80
Thyroid disorders	10	40
Epilepsy	7	28
Multiple sclerosis	3	12
Parkinsonism	3	12
Chronic renal failure	< 1	2

Table 1.2 Minor specific conditions

	Annual persons consulting	
	per 2,500	per 10,000
Acute throat infections	100	400
Lacerations	100	400
Eczma - dermatitis	100	400
Acute otitis media	75	300
Ear wax	50	200
Urinary tract infections	50	200
Acute backache	50	200
Vaginal discharge	40	160
Migraine	30	120
Hay fever	40	160
Vertigo - dizziness	30	120
Hernia	15	60
Piles	15	60

Table 1.3 Acute major diseases

	Annual persons consulting	
	per 2,500	per 10,000
Acute bronchitis	145	580
Pneumonia	4	16

Severe depression
    (parasuicide)
    (suicide)
	10
	(4)
	(1 in 4 yrs)
		40
		(16)
		(1)

Acute myocardial infarction (sudden death)	10 (5)	40 (20)
Acute strokes	5	20
All new cancers	7	28
Acute appendicitis	4	15

Table 1.4 Social pathology

	Annual persons consulting	
	per 2,500	per 10,000

Poverty
    on Supplementary Benefits
    Unemployed
	
	175
	120
		
		700
		480

Marriage, etc.
    Marriages
    Divorces
    One parent families
    Legal abortions
	
	13
	5
	40
	6
		
		50
		20
		160
		24

Crimes
    Burglaries
    Adults in prison
    Juvenile delinquents
    Children in care
    Drunken driving
    Sexual assaults
	
	40
	2
	10
	4
	5
	1
		
		160
		8
		40
		16
		20
		4

ROLES OF GENERAL PRACTICE

Within these features the GP has more general roles towards patients, practice and local community.

- For patients, the cure-care-prevention philosophies have to be applied on a personal basis, but must follow clear policies and goals.
- For the practice there have to be agreed an organisation involving the whole team with objectives, protocols, guidelines, audits and checks.
- For the community the ideals of prevention require involvement in social conditions and the environment.

The good general practice must know the availability and effectiveness of local resources. Joint experience acquired over years will enable the practice team to know who can do what for whom and how.

There has to be a build-up of experience on local hospital facilities, on the skills and personalities of local specialists and knowledge of how to obtain urgent appointments and admissions and how to match certain patients to certain specialists.

GPs have to become expert in utilising, coordinating and manipulating local medical, social and other services for the benefit of their patients.

Goals, Challenges and Targets

Accepting that we all have responsibilities for our health - GPs, patients and the community - goals, challenges and targets have to be set and met, if possible.

There are 3 areas that can be set out -

- **Clinical** good care has to be based on sound knowledge of medicine related to the special field of general practice.

- **Prevention** involves very much more than arranging for the practice nurses to carry out screening and checkups as directed by the New Contract. For success it has to have a sound educational base set up on reliable evidence that what is to be done is useful and beneficial to all. It must include primary prevention through a programme of immunisation and health education of patients with emphasis on their own responsibilities; secondary prevention through early diagnosis leading to effective treatment - this has to be opportunistic and part of every consultation, as well as in more elaborate screening programmes and checkups; tertiary prevention through successful treatment in the practice and at local specialist units; quaternary prevention must involve activation of local and national community organisations and agencies to improve social conditions.

- **Social** it is in this wider context that general practice has new roles. It has tended to restrict its interests and involvements to its own patients and practice. If the health of our people is to improve then general practice and the greater medical profession have to combine to improve the conditions and care for the more vulnerable groups of our society. This will require all GPs in every district to get together with others to define and spell out local problems and set out needs and the resources required to meet them.

If politicians and administrators are serious in their desires to improve health, then general practice and others have to produce such national and local plans.

It is wrong to expect general practice to undertake new (unproven) tasks piecemeal by direction without strategies.

Priorities

The immediate effects of the New Contract will be to alter the emphasis of work in general practice.

Figure 1.2 shows the proportion of clinical, prevention and social work in general practice in the present traditional reactive system (reacting to patient requests) and those in the newer proactive system.

Clinical work time will be reduced, and that on prevention increased.

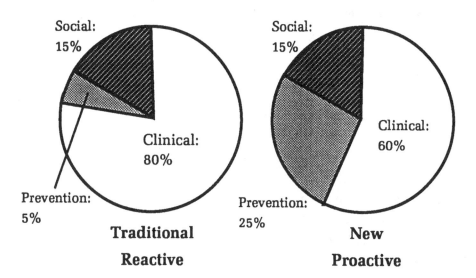

Social:
15%

Clinical:
80%

Prevention:
5%

Traditional

Reactive

Social:
15%

Clinical:
60%

Prevention:
25%

New

Proactive

Fig. 1.2 Work proportions in traditional and new systems

It has to be monitored whether such major changes will be beneficial.

New Contract

The New Contract introduces a New World for general practice. For the first time British general practice will have imposed directives, controls, checks, targets and linked incentives. The new Medical Advisers of the new Family Health Services Authorities (FHSA) will assume the mantles of highly paid local government inspectors and be expected to lay down local rules, inspect practices and issue audits.

The clinical involvement in general practice of the Family Health Services Authorities will be all-pervasive, and extend beyond the New Contract's statements and include -

- Maternity Care
- Child Care
- Family Planning
- Cervical Cytology
- Immunisation
- Prescribing
- Screening and checkups for :
    new registrants
    3 year non-attenders
    over 75s
- Health Promotion Clinics
- Minor Surgery
- Hospital Referrals
- Night Visits

In addition, there are expected to be leaflets and annual reports on practice facilities and activities.

To all this must be added seeing patients, work outside the NHS and continuing learning.

Reactions and Responses

The New Contract has been enacted.

Its contents have to be accepted and implemented.

Its philosophies are praiseworthy, but there have been no pilot trials, no tests of evaluation on their practicality and usefulness.

The ways in which it has been introduced caused much stress and anger on all sides.

...the ways in which it has been introduced caused much stress and anger on all sides.

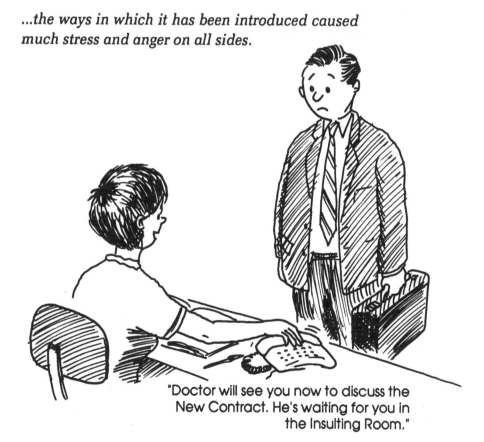

"Doctor will see you now to discuss the New Contract. He's waiting for you in the Insulting Room."

The response of general practice should be -

- Try and make the New Contract work
- Carry out co-ordinated planned evaluation and assessment of the various parts
- Produce plans of health needs for each district (or other geographical unit) for the future and publish these locally and nationally
- The response of the medical profession should be both reactive and proactive.
- However, without leadership and collaboration at all levels and in all practices and districts, little will be achieved.
- The New Contract has thrown out a challenge to the health profession. Can it meet it?

Chapter 2

Maternity Services

Good general practice is rooted in good care for expectant mothers and young children. Although almost all births now take place in NHS hospitals nevertheless the general practice team has important roles and opportunities in maternity care and then in care for infants and beyond. Good care requires good planning and organisation.

MATERNITY CARE

Facts :

- Birth rate

    13+ per 1000
    = 25-30 births per GP with 2,000 patients
    =100-120 births per practice with 10,000 patients

- Infant mortality rate (in first year of life)

    less than 10 per 1,000 births
    = 1 every 3-4 years per GP
    = 1 per year in practice of 10,000 patients

- Maternal mortality

    less than 1 per 10,000 births
    = 1 every 40 years per GP
    = 1 every 10 years in practice of 10,000 patients

- Place of birth
  99% + in NHS hospitals
  less than 1% at home or in private hospitals

- Methods of delivery
  75% spontaneous
  0.5% episiotomy
  12.5% forceps
  12.5% Caesarean section

- GP claims for intra-natal care
  10% of all births

- GP claims for shared antenatal care
  90% of all births

Aims and Policies

The aims of good maternity care are -

- Safe care for mother and child
- Personal care throughout pregnancy for mother
- Cooperative care between hospital specialist and general practice team
- Using the contacts during the antenatal period for health education of mother
- Preparation for subsequent good child care by the practice team

Common Sense Policies

Although pregnancy is a normal natural phenomenon, it is so only in retrospect. The national policy is for delivery in hospital and for shared antenatal and postnatal care between specialist and general practice teams.

Note that 1 in 4 of all deliveries involves operative procedures, caesarean section or forceps extraction. In addition
there are the extra risks of haemorrhage and difficulties with
pain control.

Most younger general practitioners will have had a period
of hospital experience in obstetrics and may consider them-
selves competent to undertake home or hospital deliveries
(in GP hospital units - where available). However, the
numbers of annual deliveries per GP (25-30) are insufficient
for maintenance of expertise.

In NHS the sensible compromise has to be -

- Shared antenatal care for all expectant mothers
- Normal deliveries by midwives who are the experts
- Abnormal deliveries by the hospital specialist team

NHS - New Contract Conditions

In the NHS general practitioners are encouraged to carry out
maternity medical services with fees for specified services.
These fees are higher for those recognised and on the
Obstetric list.

There are specific changes or recommendations in the New
Contract related to maternity services.

At present fees for maternity medical services by GP on
obstetric list are

- Complete care (including delivery) £150.00
- Antenatal care (booked before 16 weeks) £81.00
- Postnatal care - complete care £34.50
    - per attendance £4.60
    - full postnatal examination £11.50

...most younger general practitioners will have had a period of hospital experience in obstetrics...

"He specialises in Caesarian deliveries."

The annual income per GP with 2000 patients who is involved only in shared antenatal care and postnatal examination for 30 births -

- Antenatals booked before 16 weeks £2430
- Postnatal examination £345
- For a group with 10,000 patients the annual income will be £13,875

Organisation

It is useful to consider organisation of maternity services -

- What services and why ?
- How carried out ?
- Who to be involved ?
- Where and when ?

Prenatal

Prenatal or preconception counselling and advice is becoming fashionable and should be considered for a possible health promotion clinic organised and run by midwives and health visitors.

There must be more than 25-30 couples per GP considering pregnancy every year. With suitable in-practice information and advertising it should be possible to arrange group sessions which should be approved for reimbursement at £45 per session.

Antenatal

Antenatal care, shared with local hospital obstetric services, should be provided in every practice. The service is much appreciated and in addition to its clinical values it establishes and strengthens bonds and relationship with patients, involves most of the practice team and is a source of extra income.

- **How** - special antenatal clinics should be set aside. They can be run by GPs for their own patients or one or more GPs can be involved for all the expectant mothers in the practice. At each session the patient should have regular clinical assessment and also have opportunity to see the health visitor and/or practice nurse.

- **Who** - in addition to the GP there should be involved at each session the attached practice midwife, practice health visitor and receptionists - each with their own roles.

- **Where and When** - a set programme and protocol should be followed i.e. diagnosis of pregnancy, appointment for practice antenatal clinic, letter for hospital booking, completion of various forms, a two-weekly clinic should be adequate with monthly attendances in early months and two-weekly in last 6 weeks - alternating with hospital attendance. Other specials can be arranged during normal consulting times.

At least two rooms should be available, one for GP and midwife working together and the other for the health visitor who should be able to see the mother alone.

Natal

Home deliveries are rare - about 1 every 2-3 years per GP. If accepted the midwife should be in charge with GP available and in attendance when necessary.

Those GPs with hospital privileges make their own local arrangements.

Postnatal

The practice midwife will visit and attend all women delivered in hospital. There is no valid clinical reason for the GP to visit in the 12 week postnatal period unless it is considered that extra fees are required. Of course the midwife can seek further advice from the GP when necessary.

It is important that patients are taught and instructed to attend the practice children's clinic when the baby is 2-3 weeks old to see the GP and health visitor.

All women should be reminded to attend for full postnatal examination at about 8 weeks. This can be carried out either at a special clinic or during a regular consultation.

The postnatal should include a cervical smear and counselling on family planning and future pregnancies.

Self-Check Audit

As with all activities in general practice a self-check audit should be planned and undertaken with regular review and discussion by the whole practice team.

Audit requires a collection of data that can then be examined, evaluated, discussed and corrections applied, if necessary.

The collection of data is the key and the method should be as simple as possible, compatible with reliability.

For maternity care in general practice the most practical method is manual recording of each case on prepared sheets which can then be examined.

Name Date of Birth Address	Pat STILL 16.6.66 3 King St	Mary DUNN 1.7.60 Address unknown?
PARA EDD	Para-0 10.4.90	Para-2 4.5.90
ANTENATAL	Regular Attender Anxious+ Weight + Unhappy with hospital Clinic	Regular Good Coper No problems
NATAL	30.4.90 Long labour Forceps M 8lbs 10oz Unhappy with hospital	1.5.90 Short labour F 7.2 No problems
POSTNATAL	Depression Failure of breast feeding Good relations with HV	Normal Breast feeding Cervical smear inflammatory
COMMENTS	Anxious girl Afraid of another pregnancy	Follow up smear

Chapter 3

Child Care

With around 15 per cent of a practice population under 10 years of age care of children represents a considerable work load but it is important also in prevention and health promotion.

This is acknowledged in the New Contract. There are 3 parts:

- Surveillance
- Immunisation
- General Child Care

Organisational arrangements must be planned for each and all together.

CHILD SURVEILLANCE

Facts

It is evident, from the information shown in the following table, that the amount of work involved in surveillance of children 0-5 will be considerable.

	per GP with 2000 patients	per practice with 10,000 patients
Annual Births	25 - 30	125 - 150
Number of Children 0 - 5	125 - 150	625 - 750
Number of attendances for Child Surveillance		
- 1st year (4)	100 - 120	500 - 600
- 2nd year (1)	25 - 30	125 - 150
- 3rd year (1)	25 - 30	125 - 150
Total	150 - 180	750 - 900
Attendances per week	3 - 4	15 - 20

What Expectations ?

From my own practice the expected number of children who will be detected with significant abnormalities will be -

Condition	Incidence	
	per GP (2,000 patients)	per practice (10,000 patients)
Squint	1 every 2 years	1 - 2 per year
Undescended testes	1 every 5 years	1 per year
Cardiac abnormalities (all)	1 every 5 years	1 per year
Mental retardation	1 every 7 years	1 every 2 years
Physical handicap severe minor	1 every 25 years 1 every 5 years	1 every 5 years 1 every year
Deafness permanent transient	1 every 15 years 2 - 3 per year	1 every 3 years 10 - 15 per year
Spina bifida	1 every 15 years	1 every 3 years
Cleft palate	1 every 20 years	1 in 4 years
Congenital dislocation of hips	1 every 20 years	1 every 4 years
Phenylketonuria	1 every 200 years	1 every 40 years

It is important to note the relative rarity of these conditions and to realise that there will have to be very many surveillance checks to pick up such cases.

Aims and Policies

The stated aims of child surveillance are -

- Early detection of abnormalities with management to correct where possible, prevent disability and maintain optimal function.
- Development of good relations between mother-child and practice team.
- Provide support, reassurance and health education for mother.
- Ensure high immunisation rates.
- Meet the terms of the New Contract.

NHS and New Contract

Built into the New Contract are arrangements for "suitably trained" GPs to provide child surveillance service for all children 0-5 in the practice.

To receive fees GPs have to be approved by local FPCs for the Child Health Surveillance List - to be eligible they must provide evidence of having had training, experience and attended a course in the past 5 years.

A capitation supplement of less than £5 will be paid for each child for undertaking the surveillance programme including records and reports to local health authority.

WHAT, WHY, WHO, HOW, WHEN AND WHERE ?

What and Why ?

It is assumed that child surveillance is worthwhile and beneficial. There is no evidence for this. There is no evidence that the specific procedures will pick up more cases at early stages than normal practice where the mother brings the child for advice when she believes there is something "not right".

Nevertheless it is good to have regular contacts to build up good relations and teach basic elements of good child care.

Child surveillance is part of the art of sound clinical care and assessment, it should not become a stereotyped measuring exercise carried out unthinkingly.

Who and How ?

Each practice has to decide on the programme.

- What should it comprise ?

  Details should be agreed with local community paediatrician and protocol developed.

- Who should organise and carry it out ?

  Each partner for his/her own patients ?

  One partner for all the children ?

  Practice nurse and/or health visitors ?

- Is further training required ?

  Who should receive it and where ?

- What record system to be used ?

- What checks on attendances and recall for non-attenders ?

  Who should be responsible ?

- What equipment is necessary ?

When and Where ?

A special and separate clinic-session should be set aside for the surveillance programme. The numbers attending can be estimated and time set aside.

The New Contract recommends the following approximate times for surveillance examinations -

- Neonatal
- 10 days
- 6 weeks
- 8 months
- 21 months
- 39 months

To stress - one person in the practice should be responsible for organising and maintaining the programme irrespective of who carries out the examinations.

Audit Check

With the surveillance programme it is particularly important to carry out periodic checks on the "abnormality rates" and to ensure that appropriate follow-up and treatment are carried out and to assess the outcomes. All this should be entered in a separate file devoted to the programme.

IMMUNISATION

Facts

	per GP with 2,000 patients	per practice with 10,000 patients
Annual Births	25 - 30	125 - 150
Number of children 0 - 5	125 - 150	625 - 750
Immunisations (number) - 1st year of life - 2nd year of life - 5th year of life Total per year	75 - 90 25 - 30 25 - 30 125 - 150	375 - 450 125 - 150 125 - 150 725 - 750
Immunisations per week	3 - 4	15 - 20

Aims and Policies

Protective immunisation against diphtheria, pertussis, tetanus, poliomyelitis, mumps, measles and rubella is the accepted health policy in all countries. It is effective if high rates (over 90%) of immunisation are attained and maintained.

NHS and New Contract

In the NHS the GP is in the best position to achieve this programme and in the New Contract there are special incentives to reach high levels.

Highest payment will be for reaching immunisation rate for over 90% of children 12 years and less. For an average GP this will be £1800 per year.

Lower payment for 70-90% immunisation rate will be £600.

WHAT, HOW, WHO, WHEN AND WHERE ?

What and why ?

The onus and incentive has been put on GPs to provide immunisation for all children in the practice. This makes sense if complete primary health care is to be offered.

The current programme is against -

- DPT (diphtheria, pertussis and tetanus)
- Poliomyelitis
- MMR (measles, mumps, rubella)

Who and how ?

The success of an immunisation and surveillance programme lies in setting up a definite and simple scheme that can be put to expectant mothers during their antenatal period. They should be informed that they should attend the practice children's clinics as soon as they can on discharge from hospital.

Set attendance should be stated and incorporated into the various mother-held records which are provided by local health authorities.

The programme should set out attendances for child surveillance (check-up) and immunisation.

Practice decision has to be made on who is to organise the scheme, who is to be responsible for running it, checking on non-attenders and chasing them up, ordering vaccines and needles and syringes etc.

It has also to be decided who is to give the actual injections - doctor or nurse? If the latter then a doctor has to be present on the premises.

The most effective system is through the practice's own age-sex register plus records for each child to check on immunisation state plus re-checks with the FPC/health authority computer print-outs.

Where and When ?

The practice premises must have facilities for the immunisations at the times stated (usually late morning or early afternoon).

Organisation is smoother if appointments are made (and non-attenders checked) and the vaccines prepared beforehand and re-appointments made for next attendance.

...who is to give the actual injections - doctor or nurse?

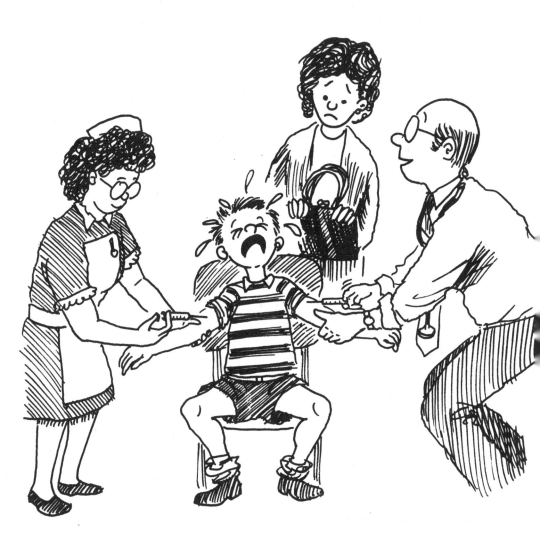

"Damn! Still, don't worry, madam. It'll be alright - we're only going to charge for one..."

The timing is under the direction of the Department of Health and the current times are -

- DPT/Polio (1) at 2 - 3 months
- DPT/Polio (2) at 3 - 4 months
- DPT/Polio (3) at 4 - 5 months
- MMR at 12-13 months
- Pre-school DT/Polio at 4 - 5 years

Audit Check

The chief concerns are to ensure -

- High rates
- Picking up and encouraging non-attenders, but accepting that some parents will decide against immunisation and their views must be accepted.
- Recording of reactions.

General Child Care

It is important to keep in perspective the priorities in child care. Whilst surveillance and immunisation are important, most important is the traditional care for children provided in general practice.

Facts - see table opposite.

Some Observations

Important in child care are -

- Knowledge of the child and family background developed over years of personal care.

- Knowledge and understanding of the natural history of childhood disorders - most recover spontaneously and completely without radical therapies.

- Knowing when child is seriously ill.

- Sensibility and sensitivity over use of modern drugs as antibiotics and anti-asthma preparations.

- Appreciation of the effects of social problems and deprivation on child fulfilment.

- Constant 'stand back' mental checks and audits to consider above points.

Facts

Annual consultation rates (per child)	
1st year	
clinical	5
surveillance & immunisation	7
total in 1st year	12
2 - 5 years	5
Annual consulting rates (children seen)	
1st year	100%
2 - 5 years	90%
Common diseases	
Respiratory & ENT	40%
Infections	12%
Skin	10%
Accidents	7%
Gastro-intestinal	6%
Behaviour	3%
Genito-urinary	2%
Other	20%
Total	100%
Social problems (per 2,0000 patients)	(families)
poverty	100
one parent families	50
juvenile delinquent	10
children in care	4

Chapter 4

Family Planning and Cervical Cytology

The New Contract makes specific conditions for cervical cytology; family planning has always been a part of general practice with reimbursement for services for the past few years.

Both are parts of the NHS preventive programme and need some planning and organisation.

Facts

- In a practice population of 2,000 persons there are 500 women aged 15 - 50 (per GP)
- In any year in the UK, 75% of women aged 15 - 50 use family planning = 375 per GP

- **Who?**

of married/co-habitees	82%
of single women	48%
of widowed/divorced/separated	55%

- **What?**

Non-surgical methods		50%
Pill	22%	
IUD	7%	
Condom	13%	
Other	8%	
Surgical methods (sterilised)		25%
Male	13%	
Female	12%	

Pregnancies (per 2,000) in one year

Births	30
Natural abortions	5
Termination	5
Total	40
Women not using family planning	85

Summary - 1 year (2,000 patients)

Women 15 - 50	500
Using family planning	375
Pregnancies	30
Abortions	10
No family planning	85

Where ?

Family planning services are available from Family Planning Clinics (FPC), general practitioners and by self-care.

	FPC	GP	Self	All
All	38	46	-	84
IUD	16	7	-	23
Condom	-	-	50	50
Other	-	-	30	30
Total	54	53	80	187 (= 50% of 375 women using non-surgical planning)

Therefore the GP with 2,000 patients can expect 53 women for family planning services in a year with income of:

46 @ £12.75	=	£586.50
7 @ £42.75	=	£299.25
Total		£885.75

Aims

The aims of family planning must be to offer advice and counselling and following consultation and discussion with the patient to prescribe the appropriate method.   Then to supervise, check and follow-up.

NHS/New Contract

It is national policy to provide a completely free (to patients) family planning service in the NHS. This continues under the New Contract. Although there are no checks carried out the GP is expected to carry out all necessary and appropriate care and service - the details are left to the GP but he/she may have to answer if there are any queries or complaints.

Organisation

The choice is between providing family planning as part of the general medical services during normal consulting sessions or at a separate clinic, perhaps associated with cervical cytology and post-natal examinations and pre-conception advice.

A Clinic is more appropriate for larger practices since the numbers of women involved would be multiples of 50, i.e. 250 a year for a group of 5 GPs. For such numbers a monthly clinic of 20-30 is feasible.

WHO, WHAT, WHERE, WHEN ?

Who ?

Although the GP is responsible, much of the work can be shared with other members of the practice team -

- Receptionists to arrange appointments and follow-up
- Practice nurse(s) to counsel and interview
- Health visitor(s) to be involved in health education and preventive care
- Midwife in the postnatal period and if interested she can also be involved in family planning.

What ?

It is evident from the tables that most of the involvement of general practice will be with general advice on the method(s) available and their pros and cons including sterilisation and termination of pregnancy, but prescribing of the contraceptive pill is the main type with insertion of IDUs also.

How ?

The practice should have some agreed guidelines on caring for women who are prescribed the pill:

- Initial checks and examinations including weight, BP, menses, pelvic examination and arrangements for cervical smear (depending on age and sexual experience of the woman).
- Follow-up - frequency, checks and examination
- Records are required. These can be those entered in the standard NHS records or on special contraceptive cards.
- Attention must be paid to ensuring completion of NHS forms to claim fees for FP Services. (FP 1001 etc.)

Audit Check

Ideally a list and records of all women receiving family planning services should be kept (list can be obtained from FPC) and tabulated so that the state of supervision can be seen at a glance. Alternatively, the information can be stored in the practice computer.

CERVICAL CYTOLOGY

Facts

- In a practice population of 2000 there are 600 women 15 - 60.
- With a cervical smear every 3 years there are 200 women at risk (but about 30 exclusions with hysterectomy etc.)
- In UK there are 2000 deaths from cervical cancer each year.
- In UK there are 4000 new cases of cervical cancer registered each year.
- In UK there are over 4 million cervical smears taken each year.
- Of these 40,000 are reported as "positive".

In a practice of 2000 there will be -

- 1 death from cervical cancer every 15 years.
- 1 new case of cervical cancer every 7 years.
- 1 - 2 positive smears every year.
- 120 smears carried out (with another 50 elsewhere and exclusions : 30)

Lives saved by cervical smear in UK = 100 a year.

Cost per smear = £10.

Cost for 4 million smears = £40 million.

Cost for each life saved = £400,000.

GP income for cervical smears per GP
- 80% target reached = £2020 a year
- 50 - 80% target reached = £734 a year

(for women 25-64 in England : 20-60 in Scotland)

Aims

The aims of the national cervical cytology programme with complete coverage of all women at risk is to reduce mortality from cervical cancer. However, there has been no significant reduction in past 10 years.

Cervical cancer is rare in general practice. The true natural history of positive smears (i.e. CIN, l, kk & lll & of inflammatory & HPV is uncertain. Therefore there is continuing debate and uncertainty on the cost-effectiveness of the programme.

NHS & New Contract

The NHS policy now is for every woman 60-64 (Scotland and England overlap) to have a cervical smear every 3 years, unless excluded.

The New Contract has changed remuneration of GPs to promote this. Instead of payment for each cervical smear carried out, now payment is to be made only if more than one half of all women at risk are "smeared" with a considerable differential to encourage high rates of 80 per cent and over. The effects have been for GPs to reduce the denominator by weeding out non-existing women 20 - 64 and so losing capitation fees and increasing denominators by encouraging attendance of these women at the practice.

Organisation

The new system of payment for cervical smears has created the biggest shake-up in record keeping and organisation.

It has meant -

- Picking out and checking NHS records for all women in this age group.
- Checking when the last smear was taken and when due for next.
- Checking practice data with those supplied by FPC.
- Inviting those due for smear to attend the practice.
- Compiling card index of all women and noting when next smear is due.
- Removing "ghosts".

(Similar exercises have been required by computerised practices)

Who ?

The whole exercise is impossible without help and input from a practice nurse and secretarial assistance. They have to prepare and check records and organise the sessions. The practice nurse should also be able to take the cervical smears and liaise with GPs in dealing with the abnormals.

What ?

The process has to be -

- Pick out those at risk in age groups who require a smear
- Send letter of invitation
- Carry out smears
- Check reports
- Follow-up abnormals
- Re-invite when next due

How ?

With more than 100 annual smears per GP it is best to organise special clinics at appropriate intervals.

Audit Check

With the aims of picking out those few women with pre-cancerous abnormalities it is important not to miss any who need follow-up.

It is necessary to have a fail-safe scheme to ensure that all with reported abnormalities are seen and dealt with either by repeat smears or referral for investigation or treatment.

Chapter 5

Medical Checks

A major base of the New Contract's clinical policies to improve health of the British people seems to be "Medical check-ups".

These include -

- Child surveillance (Chapter 3)
- New registrants
- 3-year non-attenders
- Over 75s (Chapter 6)
- Some health promotion clinics (Chapter 7)

Facts

ESTIMATED ANNUAL NUMBER	practice of 2,000	practice of 10,000
3 YEAR NON-ATTENDERS (15-74) **10% OF POPULATION 15-17**	150 (3 per week)	750 (15 per week)

ESTIMATED ANNUAL NUMBER	practice of 2,000	practice of 10,000
NEW REGISTRANTS (over 5) (removal rate)	150 (3 per week)	750 (15 per week)
POSSIBLE FINDINGS DIABETES		
known	1	5
new case	1 every 4 years	1
HIGH BLOOD PRESSURE		
known	12	60
new case	3	15
HEAVY SMOKERS (20+ per day)	20	100
OVERWEIGHT	5	25
EXCESS ALCOHOL	5	25

The estimated numbers of new registrants (5-74) to be checked and the numbers of 3-year non-attenders that will need to be invited to be checked each year are appreciable at 300 per GP with 2,000 patients and 1,500 for a practice with 5 partners 10,000 patients). For a thorough and relaxed "check-up", half an hour is a reasonable allocation of time; this means 3 hours per GP per week for the two procedures.

Aims

The presumed aims of these two time-consuming exercises are to improve health through -

- Early detection of correctable disorders and diseases
- Health promotion through advice to correct hazardous life-styles
- Improving relations between practice and patients.

It would be satisfying to those carrying out this huge volume of work to know that it was worthwhile.

NHS and New Contract

The New Contract's regulations state that -

- All new registrants to the practice, over 5 years of age, must be offered individual consultations within 28 days of registration for history taking, examination and discussion and advice to improve health. The date of invitation, the findings and conclusions are to be recorded in the person's notes. A fee of £5.80 per person is payable (approximately £870 per GP) per year on submission of claim.

- All 3-year non-attenders age 15 - 74 are to be invited similarly for a "check-up". No fees are payable.

WHAT, WHO, HOW, WHEN, WHERE AND WHY ?

What ?

For both "check-ups", i.e. new registrants and 3-year non-attenders, it is intended that attention is paid to -

- Present state of health
- Past history of important illnesses (it is unrealistic that, as this is to be carried out for new registrants within 28 days, patient's records from previous GP are not available)
- Relevant family history
- Personal risks and allergies
- Social factors such as occupation, housing, handicap, employment and income
- Life-style : exercise, diet, smoking, alcohol
- Current medication (if any)
- Status of immunisation and cervical smear
- Records of BP
        height
        weight
        urinalysis

Who ?

Except in a small practice population, it is almost impossible for a GP to undertake all this extra work alone.

It can be done if there is an employed practice nurse, able and competent, who is allocated time for this work.

Thus there should be a shared arrangement where the practice nurse organises the programme, invites, sees and checks the patients and reports findings to the GP for discussion and decisions on future care.

How ?

Organisation is time-consuming and can be complex.

For new registrants it should become the rule that appointments are given to each person to come for their check-up with the practice nurse. Prepared forms or sheets are completed and inserted into the patient's records.

For 3-year non-attenders there are major difficulties. These are, how to pick out these patients from the practice files ?

There are a number of possibilities -

- In a fully computerised practice with accurate recording of practice population by age, sex, name and address, it should be possible to programme those who have not attended for 3 years - but even here there are snags and difficulties and considerable extra expenditure.

- Manual retrospective checking of all NHS record cards for 15-74 to pick out those who have not attended for 3 years - a very time-consuming exercise, which if carried out must also include a prospective system of recording.

- Prospective recording can be achieved by flagging the card of each person 10 - 74 (10-15 year olds to prepare for the next 5 years!). The "flag" should enable the date seen and if entered in pencil this can be altered on each occasion by rubbing out and insertion of new date or by sticking on a fresh flag. Even here at the end of every year all the record cards have to be scrutinised, albeit quickly, to pick out the 3-year non-attenders.

- Another method is to arrange for FHSA to provide computerised sheets of registered person's names (age 10 - 74) and for receptionists to enter dates of every attendance or visit and then to look at these annually.

Whichever method is selected it is time-consuming, stressful for staff and costly.

When and where ?

Another major problem is that of non-compliers, non-re-sponders and non-interested. How much time, effort and money should be spent in chasing ?

How to devise convenient (for practice and patients) time and place to carry out these checks - bearing in mind that even if the practice nurse(s) are to carry out the checks they must have available room-space.

Audit Check

These medical checks, if carried out successfully, can also provide useful and valuable material for practice audits.

Records, which can be easily reviewed, should be kept of -

- Name, age, sex of all persons checked
- Positive findings
- Follow-up to see whether health advice has been followed and effective

Chapter 6

Over 75s

I nviting all patients aged 75 and over annually for consultations and advice on their health care and problems is likely to be a most onerous feature of the New Contract involving the whole practice team and requiring considerable planning and execution, but demanding above all an on-going evaluation of the exercise.

Facts

OVER 75s	practice of 2,000	practice of 10,000
NUMBERS	130	650
SEEN IN YEAR BY GP (at consulting rate of 80%)	100	500
NOT SEEN IN A YEAR BY GP	30	150
"IN TROUBLE" OR IN NEED OF REAL MEDICAL AND/OR SOCIAL HELP	30	150

NOTE : The annual consultation rate per person aged 75 and over is 7-8 per year - mean for the population is 4-5

Over 75s : where do they live ? (% of all 75s)	
ALONE	30%
WITH SPOUSE	33%
WITH FAMILY	10%
IN SHELTERED OR WARDEN ACCOMMODATION OR IN NURSING/REST HOMES	25%
HOSPITAL - LONG TERM	2%
	100%

DISABILITIES	FUNCTIONAL STATE
MINIMAL	50%
MODERATE	30%
SEVERE (housebound)	20% (5%)
	100%

MORBIDITY - DISABILITY : % EXPECTED	
VISIONS: severely restricted	10% +
HEARING LOSS : socially distressing	33% +
MOBILITY : restricted	25%
MENTAL DETERIORATION ("dementia")	20%
DEPRESSION	10%
INCONTINENCE - appreciable	5%
REQUIRING SOCIAL AIDS	33%
MORBIDITY (MULTIPLE PATHOLOGIES +)	
CARDIOVASCULAR DISORDERS (high blood pressure)	33%
NEUROLOGICAL	15%
LOCOMOTOR	25%
RESPIRATORY	10%
OVERWEIGHT	20%
FOOD PROBLEMS	40%
USING MEDICINES prescribed & self-medication	85%

Piecemeal, these tables may suggest that there is extensive morbidity in over 75s - so there is, if it is by diagnostic labelling, but functionally probably two-thirds to three-quarters are able to lead relatively independent lives with some contacts or supports from family or social services.

There are few over 75s who can be said to be completely free of any pathologies, but most can adapt and enjoy their lives.

Aims

The aims of the New Contract's proposals appear to be -

- Early detection of pre-symptomatic and symptomatic problems capable of treatment and help.
- Relief of unmet medical and social needs through available services.
- Build-up of good relations between the patients and the practice team.

Note: there is no evidence of the cost-effectiveness of such exercises.

Services required to meet unmet medical and social needs are often unavailable.

NHS and the New Contract

It is expected that all patients aged 75 and over registered with the practice will be invited every year to participate in consultations to assess their health needs.

It is stated that a written invitation should be sent out every year and this should be recorded in the patient's records. The consultation can take place at the practice premises or at home.

The consultations are to include assessments of -

- Sensory function
- Mobility
- Mental state
- Physical state (including continence)
- Social needs
- Use of medicines

No extra fees will be paid for such consultations which are to be part of the GP Contract attracting an annual capitation fee of £31.45 for every registered person aged 75 and over.

There are no NHS forms or cards to be completed or sent to the authorities and there are no indications as to how there will be checks on the scheme except the vague suggestion that the Medical Adviser may visit the practice and pick out records at random for examination.

WHAT, WHO, HOW, WHERE, WHEN AND WHY ?

For most practices this has been a new exercise and as with all the innovations of the New Contract there have been few helpful directives or examples on how to tackle the issues. Each practice has evolved its own plans of system, methods and records, and it will be fascinating to compare. As with most procedures and methods in general practice, we seem always to arrive at similar end-points and in similar ways. Nevertheless, we can always learn from each other.

Who to be seen ?

Naturally it is the over 75s and an early decision has to be made as to whether the rather illogical dictate of the New Contract is followed - i.e. to write to and invite all over 75s for a consultation or home visit, or whether the more practical procedure of using the regular consultations opportunistically for the same purpose.

For a practice of 10,000 with 650 over 75s, the costs and efforts of inviting by post and seeing them all at home or at the practice premises must be around £7000 each year if staff time and materials (postage etc.) are included.

Much better to spend some extra time, when the 80% of 75s and over who consult each year, to carry out the assessment and consultation either by GP or practice nurse.

Then, towards the end of the year, the 20% of non-consulters can be contacted and arrangements made for them to be seen or visited.

Who to Do It ?

Practice nurses have been given the tasks of organising and carrying out most of the work.

Before starting, there should be practice meetings to decide and agree on who should do what, how, and with what outcomes.

The chief aims are to pick up those at risk and in need of help and then to endeavour to arrange what is necessary.

If practice nurses are to be deputed to do the work, they must be given full support from the rest of the team and the GPs must realise that they are ultimately responsible.

What of attached health visitors and district nurses ? Their roles depend on the attitudes of local health authorities. Most are reluctant to allow their staff to do this work for GPs

- which is rather nonsensical since we should all be concerned with the benefits for patients, and these are not procedures that carry any extra fees-for-services.

Whatever the system, there should be one person responsible to the practice for overseeing and reporting.

What to Check ?

The following are to be noted and assessed according to the New Contract :

- Sensory functions
- Mobility
- Mental state
- Physical condition, including continence
- Social situation and needs
- Medication

Under each of these headings the professional who carries out the assessment should have guidelines on how each should be checked and, most important, conclusions on what actions are necessary, if any, in each individual case.

What and how to Record ?

Recording is important. It can be time-consuming and space-occupying, but both time and space should be minimal and economic.

- An up to date accurate age-sex register is essential to check on over 75s and when and whether they have been assessed.
- If opportunistic methods are used, then written invitations will be necessary only to 20% or less.

- It is essential to record in NHS records when the assessment was carried out with any relevant findings and actions to be taken.

- A special record sheet or card is essential as a check list and for recording. There are many cards and sheets (see example below), but whichever is used, they should be filed separately for reference and for each annual consultation. Any important and relevant items should be inserted into NHS records as noted above.

- Whatever system is used, any actions that require to be taken should be outlined and discussed in the practice and someone deputed to act upon them, follow up, and review.

Name:

Address:

Domicile (own home, warden, flat etc.):

Home Conditions:

Carer or nearest relative (name, phone no.):

Services involved:

Past history:

Current problems (medical, social):

Treatment / medication (current):

Last seen by GP:

Assessment

sensory functions (vision, hearing):

mobility (indoors, stairs, outdoors, housebound):

mental state:

physical (any obvious defects - BP, height, weight):

social problems (any to be taken up?):

CONCLUSIONS:

ACTIONS:

FOLLOW UP:

Audit Check

This new procedure needs to be evaluated. Therefore, each practice should carry out annual "audits" checks, reviews, analysis or whatever title is given.

Someone in the practice must analyse the records collected and report on -

- Numbers of over 75s in the practice - in age-sex register: is it accurate ?
- Numbers seen, assessed and recorded in past year
- Where seen and by whom ?
- Findings by age and sex,

    - domicile

    - functional state

    - major findings

    - actions required

    - actions taken

    - outcomes
- These can also be presented under New Contract items (under age/sex, etc.)

    - sensory functions

    - mobility

    - mental state

    - physical condition (continence)

    - social conditions

    - use of medicines

These analyses should be a regular section in the practice's annual report.

Chapter 7

Health Promotion Clinics

With "prevention" as one of the hopes for improving "health" the New Contract includes health promotion clinics as an incentive to achieve this aim. However, there is no evidence that such activities will lead to better health. These clinics are in addition to obligations for GPs to include and give in all consultations advice, where appropriate, "..... on general health, and in particular about the significance of diet, exercise, use of tobacco, consumption of alcohol and misuse of drugs and solvents".

Facts - see table on p. 243

There are numerous possible fields in which health promotion clinics might be involved. Some figures of prevalence should be noted before they are started.

These large numbers show the difficulties and uncertainties in tackling the subject -

- Which "clinics" and for what ?
- What "numbers" are copeable ?
- Where to start and when to finish ?

...there is no evidence that such activities will lead to better health.

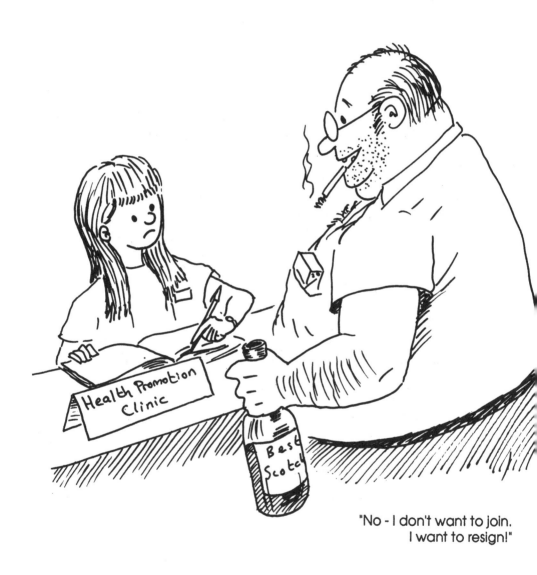

"No - I don't want to join.
I want to resign!"

SUBJECT	POSSIBLE NUMBERS	
	practice of 2,000	practice of 10,000
GENERAL		
WELL PERSONS	10-100	50-500
HEAVY SMOKERS	150	750
HEAVY DRINKERS	50	250
STRESSED	50-100	250-500
EXERCISE COUNSELLING	10-100	50-500
OBESE	50	250
SPECIFIC		
DIABETICS	30	150
ASTHMATICS	30	150
HYPERTENSIVES	100	500
CLINICAL I.H.D	50	250
STROKES	15	75
PEPTIC ULCERS	30	150
EPILEPTICS	10	50
HANDICAPPED CHILDREN (parents)	10	50
CANCERS (all) (new per year)	30 (7)	150 (35)
ARTHRITIS	60	300

Aims

The presumed "aims" of the New Contract, as noted, must be

- To promote health, hopefully
- To prevent disease through primary prevention by encouraging immunisation, avoiding risk factors etc.

    Secondary prevention through early and pre-symptomatic diagnosis

    Tertiary prevention by ensuring good management and treatment.

- To provide personal (person to person) or group counselling and advice
- To build-in an audit-check system.

NHS and New Contract

The New Contract gives examples of subjects suitable for health promotion clinics -

- Well person
- Anti-smoking
- Alcohol control
- Diet
- Exercise counselling
- Stress management
- Heart disease prevention
- Diabetes
- High blood pressure
- Post myocardial infarctions
- Arthritis

However other subjects are possible as listed in table - the local FHSA or Health Board has to approve. They will not approve any clinics for which there are already separate payments such as cervical cytology, family planning, immunisations, maternity services, child surveillance or minor surgery.

A fee of £45 per clinic is available. To receive this the clinic should -

- Be advertised to patients
- Deal with 10 persons per session, either as solo consultations or as a group (some flexibility possible by agreement with FHSA or Health Board).
- Normally last at least an hour.

Who to do What, How, When, etc. ?

Health promotion clinics are not quick and easy ways of increasing incomes. There are many and real problems.

Before embarking on the exercise there must be a practice policy arrived in consultation and discussion amongst the whole team as to whether health promotion clinics are to be undertaken and this should include assessing costs and benefits and general arrangements in the practice. Is it all worth the efforts? Which clinics? How to organise and by whom? etc.

Is it Worth the Efforts?

The income per clinic is to be £45. This may appear attractive. It is about half as much again on an insurance medical which takes 20 minutes and without any hassles.

The costs to the practice will be appreciable -

- "Advertising" and attracting patients
- Paperwork postage, records
- Staff time
- Doctor time
- Patient time
- Use of premises

It may be that at the end the "profits" on each clinic will be £10-£20, which is taxable!

What Clinics ?

The choice as noted in table - and on pages, is extensive. It is wise to begin with "simple" subjects such as well person, diabetic, asthma or obesity. The selection will depend on interests of whoever is to run the clinic and whether there is likely to be support from patients.

Who to do it ?

Someone in the practice should be in overall charge of the organisation arrangements and someone should be responsible for each clinic. It may be a GP, a nurse, a health visitor from the practice, or it may be necessary to recruit and hire (at a fee) an "outside expert" say for anti-smoking, diet or alcohol problems.

Whoever is to do it must have skills, knowledge and some expertise on the subject and also be able to run group sessions (if these are to be used). Some preliminary training may be necessary. Local health education workers are useful in these respects.

How to Attract Patients ?

Once agreed and once arrangements are ready then the clinic(s) should be advertised within the practice by notices and by word of mouth at times when patients visit the practice.

Individual invitations can also be given at times of consultation by GPs, nurse or health visitor or through the practice age-sex-disease register. Thus if a diabetic clinic is to be set up then all diabetics should be invited by letter.

What and How to Do ?

As for any form of successful education the "teacher" should prepare the work. A curriculum and syllabus should be devised along with any resources such as booklets, protocol sheets, diagrams, and audio-visual aids.

These are more important for groups than in the one-to-one personal sessions.

It is important to have help, support and contributions from the patients involved in the group clinics. Thus discussions can be led by diabetics, asthmatics etc., familiar and interested in their complaint.

Here also the local health education departments can be helpful in providing resources.

Where, When and for How Long ?

In most practices space is limited and if health promotion clinics are to be set up then an early decision has to be when can space be available ?

It is likely that out-of-hours evening sessions will be necessary and these times may be most suitable for workers and mothers.

If sessions are to last at least one hour then at least two hours have to be available on the premises. It has to be noted that whereas group sessions can easily be arranged for an hour for 10 or more persons the personal one-to-one consultations will take 15-20 minutes each and to cover 10 persons may need up to four hours.

Once started what should be done to encourage continuing attendance, but how often and for how long? It is difficult to be confident of regular continuing attendance for at least ten persons for more than say 4 monthly sessions. What should be done about non-attenders ?

Audit Check

These new methods and styles in general practice need recording, analysis and evaluation and once commenced there should be quarterly reviews on -

- Organisation and administration
- Clinic procedures
- Attendance rates
- Costs
- Benefits, if any, and for whom, and how measured.

Chapter 8

Minor Surgery

Facts

The scope for minor surgery in general practice is limited by the prevalence of "operable conditions". The table shows the estimated annual opportunities for the keen GP-surgeon (table over page).

This means that there can be two suitable cases per GP per week or over 10 per group of 5 GPs.

Aims

Presumably the intention to encourage a return of minor surgery to general practice was because it was believed that it would be cheaper for the National Health Service - this is by no means certain if all expenses are included.

For the patient, there will be a saving of waiting and travel time and enhancement of personal care by the practice team.

For the general practitioner, an incentive to increase income but also to obtain more job satisfaction and greater status and respect.

For the local general surgeons and hospital, it should mean fewer outpatient referrals and day surgery.

However, only those procedures that can be carried out safely and efficiently are appropriate, and should be confined to those listed in the New Contract; these should be done in liaison with local surgeons.

CONDITION	ANNUAL PREVALENCE	
	practice of 2,000	practice of 10,000
WARTS	30	150
SEBACEOUS CYSTS	5	25
LIPOMATA	2	10
OTHER REMOVEABLE SKIN CONDITIONS	5	25
INGROWING TOENAILS	4	20
INCISION		
ABSCESS, CYST	3	15
PERIANAL HAEMATOMA	2	10
ASPIRATION		
(JOINTS, BURSAE AND HYDROCOELE)	5	25
INJECTION		
PERIARTICULAR/ INTRARTICULAR	30	150
GANGLIA	5	25
VARICOSE VEINS	5	25
HAEMORRHOIDS	10	50
OTHERS	10	50
TOTAL	115	575

NHS and New Contract

The procedures listed as suitable and appropriate are -

- **Excisions**
  - sebaceous cysts
  - lipomata
  - skin lesions for biopsy
  - warts
  - removal of toe nails
  - intradermal naevi, papillomata, polyps
  - dermato fibromata and similar lesions

- **Incisions**
  - abscesses
  - cysts
  - perianal haematoma

- **Curettage, cautery, cryotherapy**
  - warts and verrucae
  - other lesions e.g. molluscum contagiosum
  - some naevi

- **Aspirations**
  - joints
  - cysts
  - bursae
  - hydrocoeles or epidermal cysts

- **Injections**
        intra-articular
        peri-articular
        varicose veins
        haemorrhoids
        ganglia

- **Other**
        removal of foreign bodies
        nasal cautery

- **Possibles (to be authorised by FPC)**
        vasectomy
        catheterisation
        cervical erosions
        cervical polyps
        hormone implants

For GPs who are approved and listed for minor surgery by FHSA/Health Board, a fee of £100 will be paid for each session.

A session should include at least 5 procedures, either in a single clinic or on separate occasions over a quarter. No more than claims for 3 sessions per GP per quarter, i.e. £300. A GP in a group can claim for more than 3 sessions per quarter, but the total must not exceed 3 sessions per GP.

Thus -

- Partnership of 3 can claim 9 sessions, or £900 per quarter.
- Partnership of 5 can claim 15 sessions, or £1500 per quarter

WHO, WHAT, HOW, WHERE AND WHEN ?

(Recommended reading: *"Colour Atlas of Minor Surgery in General Practice"*, Kluwer Academic Publishers, Lancaster 1990)

Note: that there is no surgery that can be considered "minor". It can suddenly turn into a major disaster either through technical difficulties or complications or sudden collapse and even death of the patient.

...there is no surgery that can be considered 'minor'...

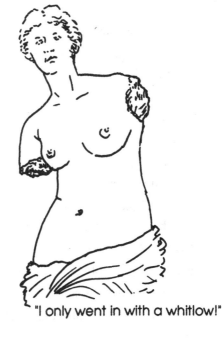

"I only went in with a whitlow!"

Who ?

All general practitioners will have had some training and experience in surgery, but some are more enthusiastic, brave and skilled than their colleagues, but even they must observe local and ethical rules and guidelines. No surgeon should ever operate alone, and his assistant, usually a nurse or colleague, must be suitably trained and experienced.

What ?

Each GP surgeon must know his/her own limitations ,and confine his "lists" to those procedures in which he is competent and safe, bearing in mind that there may be medico-legal problems if the outcome is poor.

How ?

There are basic essentials for minor surgery in general practice-

- Good arrangements and organisation.
- Adequate equipment, including safe sterilisation and resuscitation requirements.
- Good facilities in practice premises or arrangements should be made to operate elsewhere.
- Support and assistance.
- Careful preparation of patient, equipment, instruments, anaesthesia, etc.
- Patient should be given clear, simple explanation of what is to be done and how, informed of after-effects, after-care and when to re-attend.
- Arrange for histological examination of all removed tissues.
- Adhere to medico-legal requirements, such as consent.
- Keep accurate operation clinical records and an operations-book.

When?

It is best to carry out elective procedures at special operating sessions set aside for the purpose when premises will be free, surgeons and assistants unharried and unhurried.

However, it is quicker and more convenient for patients to carry out some procedures such as injections, aspirations and incisions when the patient is seen during a consultation.

Do's and Don'ts

(from *"Colour Atlas of Minor Surgery in General Practice"*, Kluwer Academic Publishers, Lancaster 1990)

DO

- Be prepared, trained and retrained if necessary
- Establish a good working relationship with your local surgeons
- Confirm medico-legal safeguards with your defence organisation and LMC
- Limit your surgery to what is feasible and safe
- Maintain accurate records of procedures and anaesthesia
- Have an operations book
- Always have an assistant
- Ensure adequate resources, equipment and facilities
- Have facilities for emergency resuscitation and staff trained to use it
- Send material removed for histological examination and swabs of infected material for bacteriological examination
- Arrange for after-care
- Acknowledge mistakes when they occur

DON'T

- Undertake what you cannot carry out safely and well ,
- Operate alone
- Work with inadequate resources or equipment
- Use general anaesthesia unless carried out by a recognised anaesthetist
- Inject steroids "blindly"
- Treat "piles" without excluding cancer or rectum or colon
- Take "short cuts"
- Be motivated by financial inducements

Audit Check

It is particularly important and relatively easy to record all minor surgical procedures carried out either in a special book, in addition to the operations book, because some will be carried out during normal consultations, or on record cards.

There should be a regular review of outcome to check on results and note any problems or complications, and take steps for improvements and prevention.

Chapter 9

Audit Checks

T he White Paper states that all doctors should be involved in "medical audit".

Audit should, and in many ways always has been, an integral part of medical practice. It is nothing new.

Good practice requires -

Questions to be asked and
hypotheses stated

Recording of data

Analysis of outcomes and
pinpointing problems

Actions for improvements

Re-checks

This is audit! It should lead to basic research studies including trials and experiments of new ideas and processes.

Facts and Critique

There are at least 4 areas to which audit can be applied.

OPERATIONAL AUDIT

- **Work in Practice**

  It is possible to determine how much work should be carried out - what is needed is to question how much is necessary and whether it is done in the best ways?

- **Practice of 2,000 persons**

  Annual consultation rate = 4-5 per person

  Annual consultations = 8,000 - 10,000
  (of these now only 10 per cent, 800-1,000 are home visits)

  Consultations per week (50-week year) = 160 - 200

  Consultations per working day (5-day week) = 33 - 40

  Consultations per consulting session (2 per day) = 16 - 20

  Length of consulting session (8 minutes per consultation) = 2 hrs 8 mins - 3 hrs.

The questions that have to be asked - are all the consultations (by a doctor) really necessary ? Some practices have an annual consultation rate of 2 per person per year and some over 7 - with apparently similar outcomes.

- **Hospital Referrals**
  It is stated that there are huge variations in referral patterns by GPs but the reasons are not so much in differences in individual habits as in the methods of data recording and analysis.

In any year in NHS -
- 13 per cent of population is admitted to hospital
- 18 per cent is newly referred to outpatient departments
- 22 per cent attend A-E departments

Translated to a practice of 2,000 patients,
- 260 are admitted
- 360 are newly referred to OPD
- 440 attend A-E department

However, it is also stated that only 1 in 10 to 1 in 20 of GP consultations involves a referral to hospital - this is quite true because there are 4-5 consultations per person which means that the denominator becomes 8,000 - 10,000 and not 2,000 !

- **Prescribing**

  The ranges by individual GP prescribing patterns are as many as there are GPs !

  PACT data is of limited value because it does not relate to

  individual patients

  diagnosis/reason for prescription

  outcomes

Clinical Audit

Logically medical audit must be concerned with the nature, course, management and outcome of disease. We know far too little about the common diseases that commonly occur in general practice.

Medical audit should include collection of data on -

- The prevalence
- The clinical patterns
- The natural course and outcome
- The management and treatment and benefits (if any) - of conditions such as -

  Acute backs

  Tennis elbow

  Rheumatoid disease

  Functional dyspepsia

  Angina

  Headaches

  Common upper respiratory infections

Hay fever
Asthma
Vaginal infections
Many others.

Prevention

It is necessary to record preventive procedures, who receives them, and with what outcomes.

- Immunisation of children should be universal and efforts made to achieve 100 per cent cover

- Immunisation against tetanus, influenza and travellers' infections requires analysis and debate
- Cervical cytology is crying out for analysis of its real usefulness and priority

- Health promotion clinics, child surveillance, health checks of new patients, 3-year non-attenders and over 75s must be exposed to critical review through audit procedures.

Social

Within all communities there are socially at-risk individuals, families and social groups. The audit procedures should aim to pick these out and to provide appropriate extra services where and when possible.

Aims

The aims of medical audit as proposed in the White Paper must be -

- To act on collected data to achieve more efficiency, effectiveness and economies in the NHS
- To use the collected data to inform and educate the public and health workers
- To define problems and weaknesses and to resolve them.

The NHS and New Contract

FHSAs (and their successors) are instructed to set up Medical Audit Advisory Groups (MAAG) composed of doctors and supporting staff. There will be funding allocated for this work.

MAAGs will be expected to -

- Institute regular systematic medical audit by all GPs
- Define problems and deal with them
- Take account of patients' views
- Produce regular reports

It is expected that MAAGs will be ready to start their work by April 1991.

Although there are many suggestions and proposals on what should be done we shall have to wait and see how successful is this ambitious scheme.

What Next ?

Audit is to become an essential part in the NHS. Its objectives are admirable, the methods and techniques need to be simple and easy but will take up time.

Audit in some form should be carried out by all practices.

MAAGs will carry out more extensive audits in each FHSA district.